Failure-Free Activities
for the
Alzheimer's Patient

*A Guidebook for Care-givers
and Families*

D1388243

Carmel Sheridan, M.A.

M
MACMILLAN

This book is dedicated to care-givers everywhere who shoulder the burden of Alzheimer's disease

First published 1992 by
THE MACMILLAN PRESS LTD
Houndmills, Basingstoke, Hampshire RG21 2XS
and London
Companies and representatives
throughout the world

ISBN 0-333-55455-8

A catalogue record for this book is available
from the British Library

Printed in Hong Kong

TABLE OF CONTENTS

NOTE TO READERS

Alzheimer's disease affects both men and women, so to simplify reading, the masculine pronouns *he* and *his* and the feminine pronouns *she* and *hers* are used in alternate chapters.

The purpose of this book is to describe activities which can bring about moment to moment satisfaction for the Alzheimer's patient. Not all suggestions will be appropriate for all patients. It is the responsibility of each reader to exercise good judgement in using the activities herein.

This book is not intended to provide medical advice and the services of a competent professional should be obtained when medical or other specific advice is required. No responsibility can be assumed by either the publisher or author for any loss or damage alleged to be caused directly or indirectly by the information contained in this book.

ACKNOWLEDGEMENTS

My thanks to the staff, volunteers and participant
at St. Joseph's Centre, Oakland, California and St
Conals Hospital, Letterkenny, Donegal, Ireland.

To the Alzheimer's Association in the United State
and the Alzheimer's Society of the U.K., for informa
tion and assistance over the years.

To Professor Martin McHugh of the Psychology
Department, University College, Galway, Ireland.

My warmest thanks to Rachel for all her encourage
ment and enthusiasm for this book

Thanks to to Bob and Eleanor for their support and
to Eddie Stack for editorial assistance.

To my family and friends for their encouragement

INTRODUCTION

For the person affected by Alzheimer's disease, the day is often filled with failures, mistakes and obstacles. These occur as a result of a reduced capacity in many areas, brought about by changes in the brain. During the early stages of the disease especially, the inability to remember and communicate things is a terrible source of frustration and stress. Without adequate memory and a capacity to know and interpret everyday happenings, the world for the victim becomes a frightening and threatening place to be. As the disease advances, the opportunity for success and a feeling of self-worth is further limited. Failure becomes an all-too-familiar experience; even in little things, the patient fails repeatedly. And every caregiver knows the frustration and helplessness that ensue.

The aim of this book is to offer simple activities which help reinforce the patient's self-esteem while relieving boredom and frustration at the same time. These activities help preserve the patient's abilities and also help to develop and use the skills he still has. The more involved Alzheimer's patients remain with the world around them, the more resourceful they become at finding ways to keep that world from slipping away.

Who Can Use These Activities

The activities described here may be used by all who come in contact with the patient: the family care-giver, the companion, the auxiliary nurse or the occasional visitor. They are described as **failure-free activities** because they are adapted to suit the needs and capacities of the person with memory loss, and are to be used in a way that will enable the person to succeed.

No special skills or qualifications are required. A gentle, caring sensitivity is all that is called for. Many people affected by Alzheimer's are aware that their abilities are fading. You must be sensitive to their deep sense of loss and frustration and do what you can to give them a sense of accomplishment and make them feel more able.

Benefits of Activities

Used appropriately, activities provide moment-to-moment satisfaction and raise self-esteem. They help nurture the person by removing the focus from the **disability** onto remaining abilities. By allowing the patient to have a meaningful role, be it dusting the furniture, shelling peas or sorting coupons, the patient's self-confidence is built up.

Care-givers can help lessen the impact of the disease by involving the patient in these non-threatening activities. They can help the patient to capitalise on whatever skills or interests are retained, emphasising assets and abilities rather than deficits.

By enabling the patient to be busy and stimulated, agitation, restlessness and problem behaviour may decrease. Involvement in activities may also keep patients better orientated to their surroundings.

Which activities work best?

Only time and experience will show which activities are the most suitable for your relative. Since there is very little evidence to suggest which activities work best, a trial-and-error approach, with adjustments based on observations, is essential.

The findings of one survey, however, may be worth keeping in mind as you set about planning activities at home. **Nancy Mace** surveyed 346 day-care centres in the United States and reported that the most successful activities with victims of memory loss were those which:

- Take advantage of old skills

- Offer social interaction
  (sing alongs, pets, visits from children.)

- Allow considerable physical activity (physical exercise, active games, walks and outings)

- Support cognitive functions (reality orientation, reminiscence, and listening to music)

Quiet games (e.g bingo) and activities requiring fine language and motor skills were found to be least successful. The survey cited the following specific activities as being most successful (those which participants seemed to enjoy most):

Sing alongs	Active games
Physical exercise	Outings
Walks	Listening to music
Reminiscence	Reality orientation
Visits from children	Visits from pets

TIPS ON SELECTING ACTIVITIES

The choice of activities is extremely important. Most patients are aware of their memory loss and failing in a simple activity will only add to their frustration. Ask yourself beforehand if the activity in question will minimize the possibility of failure and give opportunities for success.

Following are some guidelines to aid you in selecting activities:

- **SIMPLICITY**

  Use simple, familiar activities based on the person's previous hobbies, employment or life style. Patients who enjoyed cooking will still have fun mixing foods together or preparing very simple recipes such as orange juice or fresh fruit salad. Former carpenters may enjoy working with blocks of wood, nails and a hammer, while a potter might enjoy kneading a ball of clay.

  Simplicity is the key to success. Simplify the activity even further when the person seems confused by something that was previously within his grasp. The feeling of success will be retained long after the activity is over and done with.

- **FOCUS ON ASSETS**

  Use activities which draw on the person's remaining abilities and knowledge and are compatible with his level of comprehension and awareness. For example, a former handyman may have lost the skills necessary for complex jobs. But he may still be able to do simple chores around the house: jobs such as painting, sanding, washing the car and cleaning the garage.

- **REPETITION**

  Choose repetitive activities which even quite impaired patients can perform. The sense of accomplishment that comes from repetitive chores like sanding wood, polishing or dusting may be the person's only remaining source of satisfaction.

- **STIMULATION**

  As well as those activities which entertain and occupy the patient, select ones which provide cognitive and sensory stimulation and opportunities for self-expression. Reading, exercising, reminiscing and colouring are just some examples.

- **SAFETY**

  Since people with Alzheimer's have difficulty interpreting what is safe or unsafe, you must make sure that all activities are hazard-free. If, for example, the patient can no longer control sharp tools, such as scissors or knives, replace them with harmless substitutes. A plastic shovel can be used instead of a metal trowel. A wooden mallet can often be as effective as a metal hammer. Use non-toxic art supplies such as pastels, watercolours and crayons.

- **VARIETY**

  Be creative and flexible in devising activities. Add new sights, sounds and resources. Varying activities increases involvement and motivation.

  Not all activities are suitable, however. Because of the losses which accompany the disease, it's important to avoid certain activities.

Avoid Activities:

- Which require making choices or decisions. This is difficult for A.D. patients.

- Which demand any new learning. People with A.D. gradually lose the ability to learn new tasks or skills.

- Which involve attending to one thing for an extended period of time, e.g. certain kinds of craftwork or puzzles.

- Which are complex, e.g. crossword puzzles. Activities which go beyond his present skills only frustrate, confuse, lower the patient's sense of mastery.

- Which simply kill time. People in the early stages of the disease recognise worthless work and may feel slighted when asked to do it. Instead, they need expressive and useful activities to engage and stimulate them and help them retain whatever abilities remain.

USING ACTIVITIES

The activities in this book can be adapted to the unique needs and abilities of individual patients. They can be made sophisticated for someone in the early stages of the disease. Or— they can be simplified and modified as the patient's condition declines. Involvement in activities must nearly always be initiated and supervised by you, the caregiver. But be prepared to let other family members and friends stand in and take your place occasionally. This will give you time to recharge after the constant demands of caregiving.

ACTIVITY GUIDELINES

- Create a daily routine for the person. This may take some time. Don't give up too soon! In a day programme, set activities in a predictable pattern. Try to be as consistent as possible and stick to the pattern as people with Alzheimer's respond well to rhythm and routine.

- Break each activity down into small, simple steps and have the person do one step at a time. For example, in setting the table, have the patient set down the placemats first, then the cutlery, saucers, cups, plates and so on.

- Give detailed, step-by-step instructions. For example, the simple act of watering a plant involves many steps, and instructions may need to be broken down: "Pick up the jug"; "fill it with water" "pour it in here"; "that's enough" "put it down."
  If the patient receives too much information at once, he will not be able to process any of it.

- Work together in assembly line style, sharing tasks. For example, he sweeps the floor, you pick up the rubbish. He washes the dishes, you dry. He mixes the batter, you pour it into the tray. You stuff the envelopes, he seals them.

- Don't rush. Allow the patient plenty of time to do the activity.

- Allow involvement in an activity even when it seems pointless to you. Someone who is dusting a glistening piece of furniture over and over may seem to us not to be accomplishing anything. But in reality this may be a very valid way for him to spend time.

- Because the patient is unable to remember things, you can have her do the same thing over and over, day after day and still she won't get bored with it.

- Due to the nature of the disease, no activity will be successful all of the time. There will be days when nothing seems to work. Be patient and remember that tomorrow may be entirely different.

COPING WITH REFUSAL

Sometimes all your efforts will be met with resistance and the patient will refuse to take part in activities. In this event, try to role play the patient's situation. It's probable that she feels insecure and frightened about the changes taking place in her life and relationships. Saying "no" may be her only way of expressing control. Or perhaps there is simply too much noise, activity or clutter in the background. When a patient refuses to take part in an activity then, develop a mental checklist of possible reasons and go through it.

Is the activity broken down into manageable steps? Is it familiar? Are the instructions unclear or too complicated? Does the patient understand what you want him to do? Does she perceive it as childish or insulting? If any of these seems to be the problem, take steps to remedy it before inviting the patient to join.

DIFFICULTY STARTING AN ACTIVITY

Many people with A.D. find it difficult to get started on an activity. They may really want to take part but may have difficulty conceptualizing what is involved. To overcome this problem:

Show rather than tell him what's involved and then start him in motion. For example, put a paintbrush in his hand and guide him into the motion of making strokes on the paper. Give specific instructions with regard to the first step, such as "Put the brush on the paper and move it up and down" Most activities can be started in this way. for people who usually have difficulty initiating. Once started, the automatic process takes over.

If the patient still resists, try humouring him into taking part. Gentle teasing often help to defuse tension and get the ball rolling. If all else fails, you can drop the activity and try introducing it again later as he will likely have forgotten the previous experience.

DIFFICULTY STAYING WITH AN ACTIVITY

Remember that people with Alzheimer's have very limited attention spans and so they sometimes resist staying with an activity. They are easily distracted and require careful direction.

- To remind the individual to stay with an activity, simply acknowledge her presence and praise her participation. For example, "You're doing very well at that puzzle Mary, keep up the good work!"

- Use repetition: frequent, clearly stated reminders are needed to reassure the person with A.D. For example, "That's right John, dip the brush into the paint and complete the picture."

- Minimize distractions. Talk to the person in a plac that is free from distractions, such as equipmen noise, television, or other conversations. People with A.D. have very little ability to screen out distractions Keep only the material and equipment that are to be used for each particular step within reach or sight.

OTHER PROBLEMS

FRUSTRATION

People with A.D. often become frustrated. This is a ver natural response to repeated losses and failure. Whei you sense the patient is getting frustrated, drop the activity and try again later. Do this as lovingly as you possibly can. Sometimes a hug and change of subject can make you both feel better.

To minimise the possibility of frustration:

- Make sure the person is relaxed.
- Make sure she is doing one small step at a time. Breaking an activity down into small, concrete steps is essential if she is to continue doing tasks.

BOREDOM OR RESTLESSNESS

End activities when the patient gets bored or restles Don't insist on getting something done if she's not enjoy ing it or is not really involved.

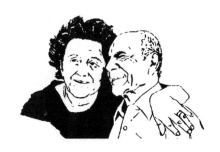

COMMUNICATING WITH THE ALZHEIMER'S PATIENT

- **Simplify communication.** Keep sentences short and explicit and avoid complicated phrases. Use the same words each time, so that the person gets used to the instructions. Keep your voice calm and at a fairly low pitch. Shouting does not help a person understand and may even make him anxious.

- **Be aware of your body language.** People with A.D. are often extremely sensitive to body language. They tune into non-verbal signals such as facial expression, body tension, mood. If you are angry or tense, they are likely to become angry, anxious, or annoyed.

- **Praise sincerely for success.** We all need to hear that we are doing a good job, and for people with dementia, this need is especially strong.

- **Slow down.** This is extremely important. You must be easy-going and relaxed. Remember the patient will mimic your behaviour. If you are uptight and too "busy", he will take his cue from you.

- **Try demonstrating visually what you are saying** The technique of doing and saying at the same time is often a very effective way of communicating. Use visual aids. Hold up the watering can when you are saying "It's time to water the plants." Support what you are saying with appropriate body language. Point to things you are talking about.

- **Never criticize.** Allow the individual to do the activity in his own way.

MUSIC

The most successful activity for people with A.D. is usually one which incorporates music. Families often comment that long after the meaning of other social cues have been forgotten, their relative still enjoys old familiar songs and melodies. In fact, the centres surveyed by **Nancy Mace** rated sing alongs as the most popular activity with victims of memory loss.

Unlike most other activities, music doesn't require a long attention span or good coordination. Since no risky materials are involved (as is the case, for example, with arts and crafts) music is also a relatively safe activity. Equally important, music is by its very nature failure-free and undemanding.

Music can be a valuable resource in recalling past pleasures. A wealth of associations, imagery, thoughts and feelings may be sparked off by a single song. Old songs and melodies are especially useful for eliciting memories and triggering the feelings that accompanied them. The familiar strains of "Silent Night" or "Teddy Bear's Picnic" are simple examples of how music can be used as an access to past experiences and events. The person will think of Christmas when she hears "Silent Night." Likewise, she will associate childhood or adolescence with "Teddy Bear's Picnic."

As well as eliciting memories, music can also stir up new thoughts and feelings. Most of the time, we listen to music for a reason: to cheer up, slow down, to relax, or to feel in harmony with those around us. Music can have the same benefit for people with Alzheimer's; moods can be created or changed. Different types of music can touch parts of the self which may be unreachable by any other means.

MAKING MUSIC

Many patients may still be able to play a musical instrument if they learned the skill earlier in life. This is because lifelong hobbies and pastimes which were always a source of enjoyment are retained the longest, even in very impaired patients. Families have told of relatives who retained the ability to play the piano well into the moderate stages of the disease.

If your relative retains such an ability, provide ample opportunity for her to enjoy it for as long as possible. Some families use music-makers such as small portable electric keyboards, which allow the patient to create pleasing sounds and also let the caregiver know where the patient is by the sounds.

LISTENING TO MUSIC

Listening to music can help a person with A.D. to reach thoughts and feelings more easily. Once you have identified the patient's preferred music tastes, you can supply appropriate background music. Tastes may vary from folk, popular, jazz, country and western, and classical to religious music. A portable "walkman" radio or cassette player with earphones may work well. Keep the music low, and try to ensure it's in keeping with the patient's preferences (no heavy rock!). Play music that evokes pleasant associations, memories, thoughts and images. If the patient is bi-lingual, music and songs from her native culture will be enjoyable.

SING ALONGS

Sing alongs can be very enjoyable for the A.D. patient and two or three people can generate enough energy for a successful sing along. Encourage the patient to hum or sing a favourite tune. Acknowledge her presence by singing her favourite song. Nearly everyone has one, even if they don't realize it! Singing a person's favourite song and dedicating it to them is a special way of saying "We're glad you're here."

- Use songs which will help to promote orientation to time, place and person. Think of all the songs you know which refer to the weather, the days of the week, the months of the year. Listening to these songs at relevant times may help keep the patient oriented.

- Select songs with place names to facilitate orientation to place.

I Belong to Glasgow	Kemptown Races
Lambeth Walk	A Long Way to Tipperary
Bonny Banks of Loch Lomond	Liverpool Lou
White Cliffs of Dover	Bladon Races
Tulips from Amsterdam	Dublin's Fair City

- Select songs with personal names—this will help to acknowledge the patient's presence.
  Here are some ideas:

If You Knew Susie	Danny Boy
Rambling Rose	Bobby Shaftoe
Ramona	Peggy Sue
O Shenandoah	John Brown's Body
Maria	Irene Goodnight
Charmaine	Daisy, Daisy

- Here are a few suggestions for seasonal songs:

Lazy Days of Summer	White Christmas
April Showers	Summertime
Those Autumn Leaves	April in Paris
We'll Gather Lilacs in the Spring	

SIGHT AND SOUND

There are some lovely video tapes available that show breathtaking scenery against a background of soothing music. If you have a video cassette recorder (VCR), you may be able to hire these tapes for a small fee in almost any video hire shop. This pleasant sight and sound method is often successful in calming a restless individual.

RHYTHM INSTRUMENTS

Rhythm instruments can be used to accompany singir
sessions. Simple instruments can be made from ordinar
easy-to-find, inexpensive things. Drums can be mac
from various containers including cereal boxes, coff
tins, or ice cream cartons. They don't have to be round

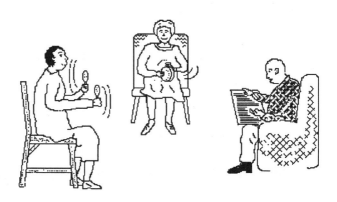

Shaking dry beans or uncooked rice in a tin will produ
an interesting sound, as will rattling aluminum foil, o
knocking wooden dowels together.

MOVEMENT TO MUSIC

Dancing or moving to music will give everyone a chan
to touch, to hold hands and get close. The patient ma
dance spontaneously to music, or with prompting ma
move to music with a strong beat—such as milita
marches and country dance tunes.

Even those who are not ambulant will find therapy i
having a care-giver manoeuvre their chairs around
rhythm to the music. Simple, gentle movements can b
carried out even with the person seated.

Following are examples of songs which are particularly suited to move to. Use appropriate motions for particular songs.

If You're Happy and You Know it Clap Your Hands

Hokey Cokey

Oranges and Lemons

Blowing Bubbles

Michael Row the Boat Ashore

When the Saints Come Marching In

He's Got the Whole World in His Hands

Do the Locomotion

The Farmer's in His Den

EXERCISE

Overall activity is often reduced in Alzheimer's disease s
that even those who were once fit and active are reduce
to leading sedentary lives. Eventually, people affecte
may become reluctant to move at all; others may pa
restlessly.

Some form of exercise should be encouraged early on
the disease to improve the patient's muscle tone ar
maintain range of motion. Exercise also helps confuse
people to sleep better at night. Perhaps of mo
importance to the care-giver is the fact that adequa
exercise helps relieve feelings of tension and anxiety ar
patients are sometimes much calmer as a result. Son
researchers have in fact shown that exercise as brief as
fifteen-minute walk has the same effect as a tranquiliz
on muscular tension.

BENEFITS OF EXERCISE

Exercise then can have both physical and psychologica
benefits, as indicated below:

- Regular exercise helps promote general fitness an
  mobility.

- Exercise reduces tension and provides a physical
  outlet for the discharge of energy.

- Body self-awareness can be enhanced through exercise.

- The patient can get pleasure and satisfaction from movement and can work through anger by physical means.

- Exercise in a group situation with family or friends can facilitate interaction and build group cohesion.

WAYS TO EXERCISE

There are numerous different ways of getting exercise. Many of these are simple methods andrequire little time and no special skills.

- At least once a day you can move the bed-bound patient's arms and legs and put her limbs through the full range of motion movements.

- When putting on a sweater, have patients stretch their arms above their head and hold this position for a moment. When putting on shoes, have them bend down and touch their toes in the process. They can rotate their hands and wiggle their fingers while watching a movie. Let them help around the house. Let them sweep, dust, mop, tidy up, fold laundry or rake leaves.

- Allow the patient to pace if she is fond of doing so. This is a common habit among those with A.D. and, although it may be annoying to you and your family, it is excellent exercise for the patient and may help tire her out by the end of the day. Leave her plenty of room to pace freely.

WALKING

If ever a fitness activity were taken for granted, it is tl
daily stroll! A recent study by the American Geriatr
Society (July, 1991) showed that a daily half-hour wa
improved communication skills of persons sufferir
from Alzheimer's disease. Walking is safe and usual
non-threatening, and you can step right outside you
front door and begin. Walking is in fact the primar
exercise for most people.

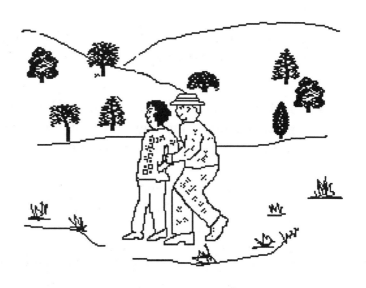

Try getting into the habit of going for a daily walk wi
the patient. Select a peaceful route; perhaps a beach ‹
quiet park. It will be easier for the confused person if y‹
go at the same time each day, use the same door and tal
the same route. Make sure both of you wear low-heel‹
comfortable shoes with an arched support. Since tl
patient may not be able to seek out experiences
stimulate his senses, it will help if you point out what l
may not be able to notice by himself: something pret

to see, to hear, to taste, to smell or to touch. Notice the sensations he seems to enjoy so you can draw attention to them again and again.

Walking can be an everyday activity, come rain, hail or shine. When the weather is poor, walking briskly indoors to the beat of music can be fun, and good exercise too! Or you can drive to a shopping complex and window shop.

ACTIVE GAMES

Physical games, simplified for the benefit of the patient, can provide a fun way to exercise for all the family. This can also be a good time for family members and the confused person to share closeness and affection without having to talk too much.

BALLOON GAMES

Balloons are soft, cheap, pretty and easy to control. Hitting a balloon back and forth is fine exercise and an excellent way to stress hand-and-eye coordination. A number of simple games can be adapted to suit the ability of the patient.

- For active patients, a net can be set up and a game of balloon volleyball played.

- For a group game in the home or nursing home, players form a circle and the balloon is batted at random from one person to the next. It is kept circulating for as long as the energy lasts.

PASS THE BALL

A simple game involving three or four people. Players sit or stand around in a circle at arm's length from each other. The leader hands the ball to any one player and asks him to pass it to a person on either side. While passing it, he says the person's name. The ball is passed around from person to person for two to three rounds.

RING BOARD

Rings was a popular game in bygone days. Ring boards are available in sports or toy shops or you can make your own by screwing large cup hooks into a piece of plywood. Hang the board on a wall and show the patient how to toss the rubber rings at the hooks.

CATCH THE BAG

This is a simplified version of the usual "Catch," suitable for two players. Instead of using a ball, a small bean bag is hung from the ceiling and swings back and forth between two players. This is also an enjoyable activity for young people and it can be played while seated.

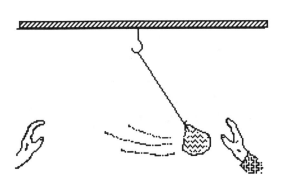

BOWLING

Bowling is a wonderful failure-free game which can be played by arranging plastic skittles or ten pin bowls on the floor. The ball is rolled to the patient who aims for the pins. This is a useful game for exercising the arms and trunk since the player must bend to catch the ball and flex the muscles to roll it to the pins.

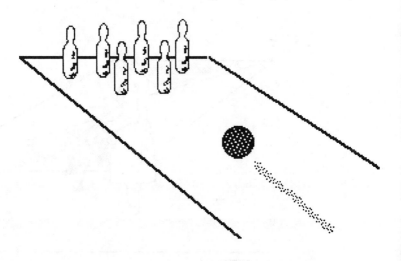

Bowling can also be played by arranging skittles on a long table of suitable height. A trap for the ball can be made at the end of the table.

If the patient is wheelchair-bound, a simple cardboard guide can be made to rest on her knees so that she can roll the ball down the guide towards the skittles.

SHUFFLEBOARD

In this game, small wooden discs are pushed with
a shuffleboard stick as far as they can go on the
shuffleboard base. Shuffleboard is an ideal out-
doors lawn game for sunny summer afternoons.
The entire kit, including the sticks and wooden
discs may be made quite easily. The base can be
made from heavy linoleum or plastic and marked
into segments.

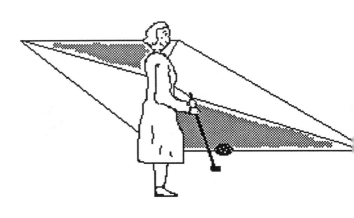

BASKETBALL

A simplified version of basketball can be played
where the patient tosses a rubber ball into a

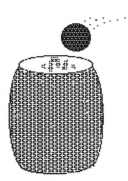

laundry basket. The care-
giver retrieves the ball after
each pitch and rolls it back
to the patient.

CIRCLE TOSS

Three concentric circles are marked on a board, large piece of plastic or cardboard, which is placed on the floor. The patient sits or stands outside the outer circle and tosses three beanbags at the bull's-eye which is the inner circle.

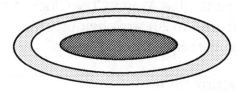

BEANBAG TOSS

Prop a heavy board with large cut-out holes against the wall. Ask the patient to throw a beanbag into the holes. This activity can be done from a sitting or standing position.

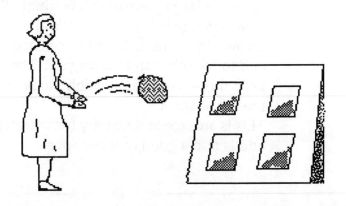

DARTS

Playing darts can be fun and safe. Never use darts with steel points, only those with suction cups. When they hit the metal target they adhere to it. Velcro dart boards with Velcro covered balls are also widely available at toy stores now. When playing darts, remember to keep the game simple—games like Around The Clock (hit the numbers from 1 to 20), are obviously much better than a game requiring arithmetic.

PENNY PITCH

Each player gets ten pennies. A shoe box is placed five or six feet away from all players, and the players try to toss their coins into the box. When they succeed, everyone cheers. A small token prize may be given to whoever gets most coins in the box.

PARACHUTE TOSS

This is a good group activity and ideal for exercising and using eye and hand coordination. Patients grab the edges of the parachute (a sheet can substitute or a large piece of fish netting). Beach balls, small sponge balls, punch balls and balloons are thrown in the middle and tossed about from one end to the other and back again. The object is to keep those round lightweight items from leaving the net or sheet.

This is an excellent activity for wheelchair patients and is also a good outdoor sport.

DOMESTIC EXERCISES

Taking part in household chores can give the patient a
chance to exercise and a sense of doing something
useful. Ideally, you may be able to establish a routine of
household activities based on what was enjoyable in
the past. Select chores which are relatively simple,
repetitive and hazard-free. For example, at mealtimes
perhaps the patient could contribute by:

- Handing out paper napkins
- Putting out the placemats
- Sorting and putting away cutlery after meal

Repetitive actions are a common characteristic of A.D.
behaviour. You can capitalize on this pattern by
selecting household activities which involve repetitive
movements. These should be simple enough to be
completed by the patient. Remember it isn't so important that the job be done perfectly—but it should give a
sense of accomplishment to the patient.
Here are some ideas:

Raking leaves	Picking up fallen fruit
Dusting	Mixing batter
Vacuum cleaning	Shining shoes
Mowing the lawn	Scrubbing potatoes
Mopping the floor	Tearing lettuce leaves
Whipping cream	Sanding wood
Beating eggs	Sorting laundry

LIGHT BODY EXERCISE

Confused people often enjoy doing light body exercise as part of a group or with a partner. When you try these exercises, teach each one by demonstration and have the patient imitate what you do, gently guiding him if necessary. If he has arthritis or any other medical condition that makes movement a problem, ask a physical therapist to recommend special exercises for him.

To minimize confusion, try to exercise at the same time each day for about ten minutes and follow the same sequence of activities. Start from the head and work all the way down to the feet, beginning with a gradual warm-up to loosen tight muscles. Light rhythmic clapping and stamping are good warm-up exercises.

Begin with the upper body.

HEAD AND NECK

- Look straight ahead

- Bend ear to shoulder and hold

- Repeat for other side of body

FACE

- Give a broad smile— show your teeth

- Raise your eyebrows

- Pucker your lips— kiss

- Blow out a mouthful of air

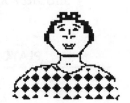

SHOULDERS

- Raise shoulders up to earlobes—
  shrug

- Relax shoulders

- Repeat

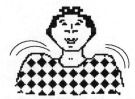

ARMS

- Stretch both arms straight in front.
  Hold palms up.

- Move arms upward as far as possible

- Lower arms slowly to lap

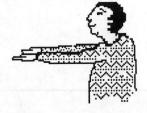

HAND EXERCISES

Hand and arm exercise can be achieved through rolling playdough and tying simple knots. Both activities should aways be supervised.

PLAYDOUGH

- Show the patient how to shape playdough into a long roll.

- Then roll it back and forth, from palm to fingertips

- Fold it in half and repeat the preceding steps.

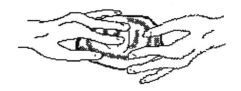

TYING

- Tie and untie simple knots in soft cord and encourage the patient to copy you.

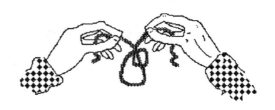

CHAIR EXERCISES

The following are a few simple exercises which can be done from a sitting position. Begin slowly, asking the patient to imitate you

UPPER BODY

- Sit upright and spread knees

- Slowly bend forward from the waist

- Reach hands toward floor and hold for a count of two

- Slowly return to straight position

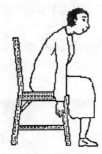

LEGS

- Place feet flat on floor

- Raise one leg in front as far as you can

- Hold for a count of two

- Return foot to floor and relax

KNEES

- Place feet flat on floor, and arms by side

- Bend knee and raise foot slightly from floor

- Return foot to floor

- Repeat with other leg

FEET

- Place feet flat on floor

- Lift one foot off the floor, then the other Stamp gently in marching fashion

- Place both feet on floor again and relax

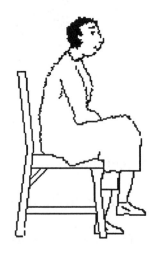

Conclude exercise session with a slow stretch to cool down—

- Sit straight with arms on lap

- Slowly raise arms above head and take a deep breath

- Slowly lower arms and exhale

- Relax

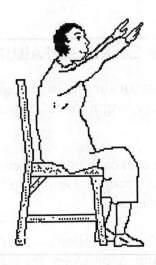

EXERCISE TO MUSIC

It is often helpful to exercise to music and use props such as balls, wooden dowels or elastic ropes. Both music and exercise involve rhythm, tempo and movement. The rhythm and tempo of a piece of music may help cue the timing and pacing of movements such as leg lifts or stretches. Swaying to music, clapping hands or tapping feet are all simple exercises which stimulate the flow of oxygen to the brain.

Use soft background music which will not interfere with the patient's ability to hear and process your instructions. Have him imitate what you do and if he gets stuck or has trouble, try helping him move gently.

MAKING EXERCISE FAILURE-FREE

- Begin with simple, easy-to-follow exercises and limit the length of time spent at each to five minutes.

- Move into each new exercise slowly. Monitor the patient's progress and stop if he seems to tire or lose interest.

- Simplify instructions —don't give directions which distinguish between the right and left sides of the body.

- Avoid using exercises which require the patient to hold his breath too long or stamp his feet energetically as these will cause strain or overexertion

- Stop and rest after every five minutes or so and have a conversation with the patient. Talking and having fun will make an activity more enjoyable and double the benefit.

- Watch for signs of overexertion. Suggest that the patient slow down if he seems to be overdoing it.

FOOD PREPARATION

Many Alzheimer patients are able to do simple food preparation, and all are adept at sampling the finished dish! Day care centres often find that simple cooking activities are well within the grasp of Alzheimer patients. Women generally respond especially well to this activity, probably because food preparation has been a large part of their active lives. Memory of this involvement is stimulated through sight, sound, smell and taste. At the same time, this activity emphasizes sequence, counting and object identification.

MAKING SESSIONS FAILURE-FREE
Certain precautions must be taken to make this activity both failure-free and hazard-free.

- Each task must be broken up into its smallest components and continuous direction given on each step. For example:
  "Break the eggs—now beat them."
  "Wash the vegetable—now slice it."

- The exercise should also be quick to complete because of the patient's short attention span.

- As few ingredients as possible should be set out at any one time, and the patient should be familiar with those used.

- Examine activities for potential hazards before beginning. Sharp instruments should be put out of reach.

- If an activity calls for tinned ingredients, tins should be opened by the care-giver. The contents should be put into a bowl and the container thrown away.

- On no account should the patient be allowed to use a stove or barbeque.

ACTIVITY IDEAS

BISCUIT BAKING

With some supervision, biscuit baking is an activity well within the grasp of many patients. Using a favourite biscuit recipe, jobs can be assigned on the basis of the patient's ability. Specifically, ingredients must be measured, sifted, beaten together, and the uncooked biscuits put on baking trays.

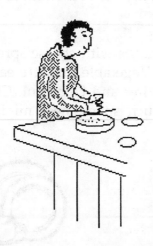

SALADS

With your assistance, the patient may be able to help prepare a full salad such as cold meat, vegetable, fruit tuna or salmon. Whatever type of salad is being prepared, the same basic steps are involved. The patient might assist in washing the lettuce and other vegetables, and tossing the salad with dressing.

CAKES

Cake decoration can bring almost immediate gratification because of instant colourful results. The patient may be able to help mix the icing, colour and flavour it, and put the decorations on top of a ready baked cake. Cakes can also be baked quite easily using cake mixes which just need water, milk or eggs

DESSERTS

Various desserts can be made using assorted tinned or fresh fruit and served with whipped cream or yoghurt. Pastry shells filled with fruit and covered with topping make an appetizing dish. Dessert which only need cold milk can be served up with jelly

SNACKS

Sandwiches with cheese spreads can be made quite easily. Vegetable dips are easily prepared and look appetizing and colourful. Cheese and biscuits and other such snacks need minimal preparation.

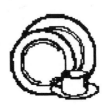

SIMPLE RECIPES

You will find simple recipes in cookbooks, magazines and newspapers which can be adapted to involve the patient in some or all of the steps in preparation. Again, the level of involvement will depend on the patient's capabilities. Supervision is very important and hob and oven procedures should only be carried out by the care-giver.

The following recipes are quick and easy to prepare. You can compile a programme of simple recipes of your own.

KEDGEREE

This is an interesting recipe which tastes delightful and can be made quite easily. You will need the following ingredients and the rice and eggs should be prepared in advance and allowed to cool. The fish should be drained and left on a plate. The patient will be able to wash the vegetables and maybe prepare them under supervision. To prepare the dish you will need a large bowl and wooden spoon.

6oz. /200g. cooked rice.
1 tin of salmon or tuna, drained
Half a chopped green pepper
Half a chopped red pepper
3 spring onions, chopped
1 tomato cut in wedges
2 hard boiled eggs
8 tbs. /half a small jar mayonnaise
seasoning to taste

The ingredients are mixed together in a large bowl i
the sequence listed above—first the rice, then fisk
peppers and so on.When the kedgeree is thoroughl
mixed, it is chilled for an hour or so. Served on a be
of lettuce and garnished with chives and lemo
wedges, this dish also gives the patient good involve
ment in the presentation and serving activities.

NUTRITIOUS PEANUT BUTTER SNACK

You will need the ingredients below and a large bow
and wooden spoon for this recipe.

8 oz. /250g. peanut butter
1 tbs. margarine
4 oz. /125g. nonfat dried milk
3 oz. /100g. chopped nuts
3 oz. /100g. raisins
4 oz. /125g. dates
4 oz. /125g. digestive biscuit crumbs

The care-giver should soften margarine and mix wit
peanut butter while the patient is crushing biscuit
into crumbs. Then the softened mixture and dried mil
are mixed thoroughly in the bowl by the patient. Ra
sins, nuts and dates are added and mixed. The mixtur
is shaped into little balls by the patient and rolled in th
digestive biscuit crumbs.

FRUIT COMPOTE

This is a simple dessert to prepare and you can vary the fruits to suit tastes. It is served with whipped cream which the patient can prepare. The care-giver should open the tin of pineapples, put the fruit on a plate and save half of the liquid.

Seedless white grapes
A crisp apple
Pineapple chunks
2 Satsumas

The patient can peel the apple and maybe dice it under supervision, peel the satsumas and separate them into segments. Then the grapes, apple and satsuma are mixed together with the pineapple juice. The fruit compote is chilled and served topped with whipped cream.

CRAFTS

Craftwork is a creative activity and forms an integral par
of many activity programmes in hospital and day-care fa
cilities for elderly people. With proper planning and
safety measures, craftwork can also be a therapeutic and
enjoyable activity for the patient at home. As with other
activities, crafts should be chosen with the capabilities o
the patient in mind.

- Crafts are suitable only for the person who can
  concentrate long enough to be able to follow the
  sequence of steps involved.

- The craft project must be carefully selected.
  Specifically, it should be simple enough so it will be
  completed by the patient rather than by the care-
  giver.

- Crafts which entail only a few large, easily
  manipulated components work best.

- It is important that the project be quick to
  complete. Otherwise, the patient will become
  restless because her attention span is limited.

- Only crafts which are adult in kind should be
  attempted since making fun figures or other
  childish objects will do little to raise the patient's
  self-esteem.

- Abstract projects should be avoided since they will be outside the patient's range of comprehension. The patient will be better able to relate to a structured project with well defined steps.

- It is helpful to have a ready-made model object which the patient can see and examine. This will help him visualize or imagine the end product. Introduce the steps involved one at a time. Keep in mind that even with a demonstration and ready-made model, there is no guarantee that a similar finished product will always materialize. It is in the **doing** that fulfilment occurs, rather than in the end product of a project.

MAKING CRAFTWORK HAZARD-FREE

The patient will need continuous supervision during craftwork. He may lose the ability to discriminate between what is and what is not edible, so it is essential that all materials used be nontoxic. The care-giver must scrutinize projects thoroughly to check that all possible hazards are eliminated. For example:

Does the project involve the use of small objects such as coins, marbles or buttons? Is the patient prone to putting things in his mouth?

If so, this information must be made available to all those involved in activities so that risk can be eliminated. Patients who are allowed to work with materials such as needles, scissors and glue must be able to use them appropriately and even then, they must have supervision.

COLLAGE IDEAS

Making a simple collage involves gathering magazine selecting pictures, cutting them out, and arranging an pasting them on blank paper. This is a most suitable cra activity for the A.D. patient because it can be broken int separate, simple steps and requires little effort or skil Collage-making is also a relatively clean and quie activity which can be an individual or group project.

Treasure old magazines since they are full of collag material. Search through them for pictures that will hel illustrate a particular theme. Gardening and cookin publications will provide a supply of colourful picture: Under supervision the patient can cut these out and stor them in a box specially for collage materials. To make th collage, the patient selects pictures of a certain theme an arranges them on a sheet of paper or cardboard.

SEASONAL COLLAGE

This collage will help reinforce awareness of tim and year. An Easter collage in the springtime colours of green, yellow, pink and lavender can be made quite easily just from pictures. Seasonal themes also provide good conversation material fc the patient. Travel brochures, calendars and advertisements are ideal sources for summer, autumn or winter collage pictures.

EVENTS COLLAGE

The "event" themes are endless. Weddings, births graduations, and moving house are some of the special events which may be significant to the pa- tient. The event can be assembled from colourful pictures into collage form.

FOOD COLLAGE

A collage of favorite foods can be made quite easily by pasting or taping colorful magazine pictures onto heavy cardboard.

PEOPLE COLLAGE

This collage could be of famous people, people working in different occupations, people involved in different sports, or playing different musical instruments. It might be a collage of people from different places. The possibilities are many and varied. A places collage is also a nice project. Be creative!

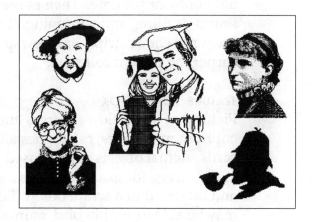

SCRAPBOOKS

Scrapbooks centering on various themes may be mad quite easily and will give many hours of enjoyment afte completion. Magazines, newspapers, cards and phot graphs are good sources for pictures.

FAMILY SCRAPBOOK

Mementos of family celebrations such as births an weddings, and pictures of places lived in can form the basis of a family scrapbook. This will also be a good memory prompter for the patient.

HOBBY SCRAPBOOK

Special interest magazines can provide many colourful pictures for a scrapbook devoted to an old hobby or pastime. Themes may include sports, stamps, sailing, and gardening. It might even be favourite comic strips, or a newspaper recipe corner the patient collected.

NATURE SCRAPBOOK

Pictures of birds, flowers, trees and animals may b cut from magazines, catalogues and Christmas cards. Actual objects may be used where appropri-ate; flowers, for example, can be collected, presse and mounted in a scrapbook. Wildlife associations may be able to supply bird, animal, tree, and wild-flower resource books for nature scrapbooks.

SEASON'S BOOK

A special book may be started at the beginning of the season. Here the patient can be helped to record dates of special outings, family activities, etc. Photographs may facilitate recall along with mementos like ticket stubs and programmes.

CRAFT IDEAS FROM OUTINGS

The patient can record outings through simple craftwork. As well as providing fun and therapy, these projects may also help the patient to remember the outing.

MOBILES

A woodland mobile can be made from leaves, horse chestnuts, pine cones, pebbles, sticks and other small specimens collected on a journey out of doors. These simple nature materials can then be tied to a clothes hanger with different lengths of string, thread or wool.

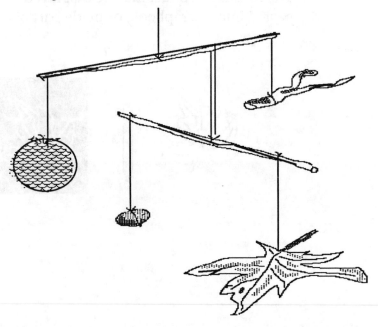

Alternatively, the woodland specimens could be stuck to wide masking tape and hung from any kind of rod.

RUBBINGS

Rubbing is similar to tracing except that the finished design is more shaded, and has a slightly three dimensional look. Here are a few things that take rubbings well: leaves, engraved signs, coins, the bark of a tree. Greaseproof paper or tracing paper can be laid over the object to be rubbed. The texture can be recorded on paper by rubbing back and forth over the textured surface with a pencil, crayon, or chalk.

The finished product may be displayed on a door, pasted into a scrapbook, or made part of a collage.

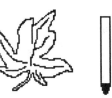 

GARDENING

Gardening has long been thought of as a healing or therapeutic activity. In essence, it involves caring for a form of life and creating something of visual beauty. Since gardening stimulates memory through the use of all five senses—seeing, hearing, smelling, touching and sometimes tasting, it is well suited to the person with memory loss.

Select gardening activities which will require just enough attention for the patient to feel occupied, without becoming tired or feeling tied down. Everyday chores such as mowing the lawn, leaf raking and weeding can be done easily enough with some help and supervision. But keep in mind that if the work takes too long and becomes overwhelming, it loses its therapeutic value. Here are some ideas for simple and creative gardening projects.

PLANT A TERRARIUM

When a clear plastic or glass container is filled with soil and plants and covered to form a miniature landscape, it is called a terrarium. Easy and inexpensive to make, the terrarium will add a pretty touch to the patient's room and give her something pleasant to look at. When friends visit it will make a fine conversation piece as it is such a novelty and tends to arouse curiosity. The terrarium when finished takes on the major responsibility for controlling its interior temperature and keeping the moistu level constant. The rest is up to you and the patient.

PLANTS

Decide on the plants you want to grow in the terrarium. You can plant a woodland, desert or flower-garden. Just keep in mind the full-grown plant size, how it grows, and where it likes to grow.

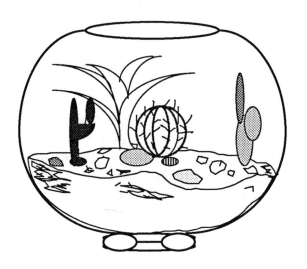

CONTAINER

Select a container, preferably one of clear plastic and as close to colourless as possible. The most common terrariums are planted in unused fish bowls, brandy snifters or apothecary jars. The mor unusual the container, the more intriguing the ter rarium will be.

Involve the patient in turning the terrarium about once a week and in watering it very occasionally.

WINDOW BOX FLOWERS

Flower boxes are very attractive and like terrariums, they are easy to care for. The patient may be able to help select the seeds and tend to the flower box once sown. Even the patient who is wheelchair-bound will be able to tend the window box flowers if they are within reach.

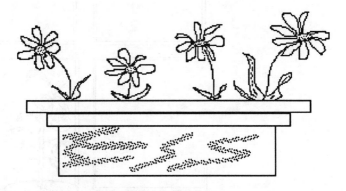

* Decide on the flowers you want to grow. Your choice will depend on window exposure, room temperature and the space available. Start your flowers from seed or buy bedding plants. Once the plants are in place, put a layer of moss on top of the soil to keep it moist and cool.

* Use a memory aid to remind the patient when plants need watering. A 3 x 5 index card with large, clearly typed instructions will be useful along with prompting from a family member.

* Encourage the patient to touch plant leaves and flowers. The smooth feel of a rose petal can give a little enjoyment. Feeling the texture of the soil or the tenderness of the seedling can bring pleasure.

INDOOR VEGETABLE GARDEN

Try raising a plum or cherry tomato plant in a large flower pot—it works! Keep the plant in a sunny spot for as long as possible. Have the patient water it thoroughly every day. When the plant is about ten inches tall, stake it and keep it trained to the support while it grows.

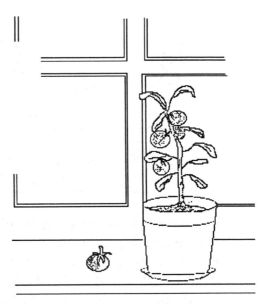

SPROUTING SEEDS

Involve the patient in sprouting seeds like alfalfa and mung beans. These grow visibly every day and can be eaten in salads and shared with others.

INDOOR HERB GARDEN

You can grow lots of fresh herbs on a bright kitchen windowsill all year round. As well as looking nice, herbs smell good and will make the room feel clean and bright. They will provide a focus for the patient and stimulate the senses. Like the terrarium, the herb garden is sure to make a fine conversation piece. It does well with very little care which the patient can give with some supervision and prompting. A memory card with instructions printed in large type should be left by the herb garden.

- Basil, dill and rosemary are three herbs that can be easily grown from seeds or bedding plants. Use separate clay pots for each individual herb with its name clearly marked on it.

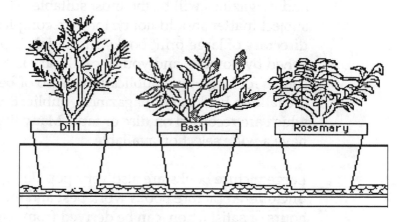

- Put the pots into trays holding about an inch of pebbles. Pour in just enough water to cover the pebbles. Place the tray on a sunny windowsill.
  Have patient water plants daily and turn the pots one-quarter turn.

SOLO ACTIVITIES

Solo activities can be designed so they demand little inp
from the care-giver. They are ideal to keep the patie
occupied while the care-giver attends to other tasks. Li
many other activities, they are so simple that they a
often overlooked.

READING

If the patient is still able to read, large-type books
and magazines will be the most suitable. The
subject matter should not be long or complex. A
directory of large print books and serials is published by Bowker, and your local library is a good
source for large-type publications. Also of benefit
are talking books and magazines, publications
which are recorded on disc or tape. Many librarie
have a wide selection available.

Large picture books are also very popular. Simpl
uncluttered picture books work best and many
hours of satisfaction can be derived from scannin
the pictures of popular children's books. Collecti
books of famous comic strip characters can also
provide quiet enjoyment.

TELEVISION

Some patients still enjoy watching TV even though they may have difficulty following the story-line. Others may find television threatening and so it is important to monitor viewing.

By observing how the patient responds to various programmes, you will be able to chart what is suitable and stimulating for her. Action-packed programmes are best avoided.
If used correctly, TV can become a useful resource and be of benefit to the patient. As well as its entertainment value, television has much potential for rekindling old interests. A lifelong interest in classical music, for example, may be restimulated by viewing concerts or ballet. Someone who had an interest in athletics may have this interest revitalized by watching sports. The most popular programmes tend to be :

    (1) Comedy

    (2) Children's educational programmes

    (3) Wildlife and sports

WINDING

Winding a ball of wool or a spool of thread is an activity well within the grasp of many patients. Unravelling old knitted garments is also an activity which many families find popular.

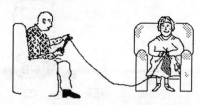

SHELLING

One care-giver told of her relative getting long periods of satisfaction from shelling nuts. Friends brought bags of nuts to be shelled, so the task coul be carried out to the benefit of the A.D. patient an the visitor! In this activity, provide a small bowl for the shelled nuts and another for the shells.

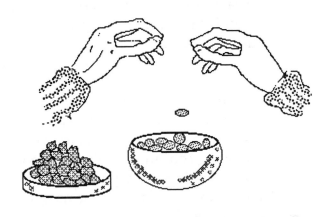

SORTING

Sorting buttons according to shape, size or colour and putting them into bags can be a useful activit Some patients may be able to sort them accordin to material, with metal, plastic and cloth ones bei tipped into separate jars. This activity must be carefully supervised.

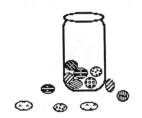

Coins of different denominations can be sorted and put into separate jars. This activity can keep the patient engrossed while at the same time offering a service to you.

There are endless ways in which old keys may be sorted: the thick ones separated from the slender; the long from the short.

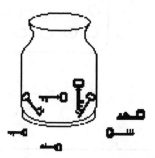

Playing cards may be sorted according to numbers, colours or suit. Postage stamps may be sorted for charity.

Encourage the patient to help you sort and match clothing before and after your weekly laundry. Perhaps he can help you separate white and dark colours, or maybe sort clothing according to fabrics. When the wash is done, the patient may be able to help out in sorting clothes of all different sizes and in matching and pairing socks. There are many other simple household tasks that involve some element of sorting which the patient may be able to carry out.

LACING

Simple lacing kits are available which can provide quiet activity.

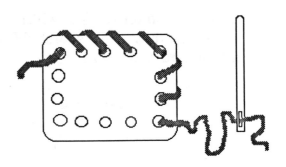

STRINGING

Large coloured wooden beads or blocks can be strung on a piece of wool. A kit for this activity will include ready-to-string coloured pieces and some wool.

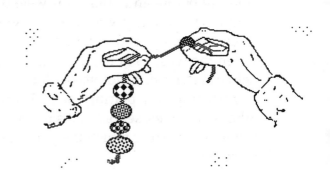

TEARING

Some care-givers find that computer sheets with the perforated tracks on the side make an engaging activity. The patient will sit for hours and tear off the edges.

WORKBENCH

Many patients enjoy working with miniature workbenches which have large plastic screws and bolts. They can screw and unscrew the bolts. Others enjoy taking to pieces items such as old radios or doorknobs.

DRESSING CARD

A dressing board can be made quite easily. Attach to the board such things as a button and button-hole, a zipper, a hook and eye, a door knob, a padlock with a key, a snap fastener, shoestrings, and a slip lock bolt.

Working with such items offers motion rehabilitation for pushing, twisting, pulling, turning and sliding.

ACTIVITY APRON

Activity aprons are available which help keep the busy fingers of the Alzheimer's patient meaningfully occupied. These aprons are covered with things to touch and manipulate: buttons, beads, zippers, pockets, Velcro fasteners and ribbons to plait.

SOLO GAMES

It is easy to adapt some children's educational games t
suit the Alzheimer's patient. As with all activities, sol
games should be geared to the patient's capabilities. Th
games should not be complex and should have larg
components. Games with the following themes may su
the patient and similar versions of them are availabl

MATCHING

A series of cards are assembled to form a matching
activity. Here, simple objects that relate to each
other can be paired off, for example, a dog with a
bone or a telephone with a receiver. Or, as in the
examples below, two cards can be matched to form
a single object.

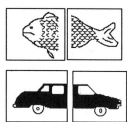

You can also make your own matching cards.
Again, look to magazines for pictures and ideas.

SEQUENCE CARDS

A series of cards can be arranged in sequence to tel
a story, each scene being made from 2 or 3 sequenc
cards. Themes for sequencing games are numerou
and the game has a short attention demand which
makes it suitable for Alzheimer's patients.

PEGBOARDS

Working with pegboards helps to develop fine motor control. There are many varieties of pegboards available. The most suitable pegs are those which are large and easy-to-handle and have a shoulder which gives a positive stop and helps them fit snugly into the pegboard.

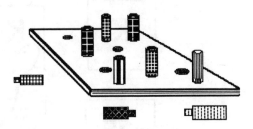

SHAPE PUZZLES

These are games where a number of plastic or wooden shapes are fitted into corresponding holes in a board. They can spark off a discussion on shapes: squares, triangles, circles, e.g. *"Show me another triangle." "Point to the two circles."* Colours can also be discussed, e.g. *"Find another the same colour as this—What else is green?" "Have you any clothes the same colour as this?"*

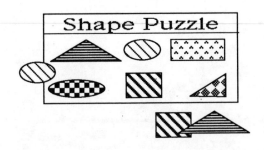

LOTTO

You can make lotto games quite easily using a larg
piece of paper or cardboard as your lotto board.
Trace about six squares on the lotto board and stic
on pictures. Mount similar pictures on stiff cardboard pieces for matching.

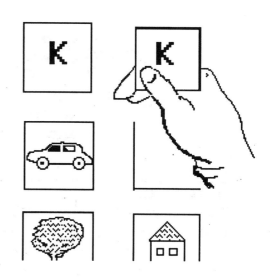

ART

Simple art activities provide creative opportunities for self-expression. Inexpensive adult art supplies can be obtained at most art supply stores. Crayons, soft pastels, oil pastels, finger paint and felt-tipped pens are all you need. They are essentially failure-free as they move easily and quickly.

Let the patient know he doesn't have to be an artist and he doesn't have to make anything. You might have to start him off especially if the process is new to him. Be sure to make no demands and never make corrections. Encourage him as he works. Give praise often and freely. Ask him to talk about his picture. Say, for example, "Tell me about your picture" "What's the story?" "How does it make you feel?" Don't attempt to interpret the meaning of someone's art. Supervise art work closely as the patient may mistake rinse water for drinks or clay for food.

WORKING WITH COLOUR

Colour is a symbolic language which can help people express their emotions. Drawing and using water colours gives good opportunities for self-expression. There are many adult colouring books on the market now which feature interesting outlines for people to fill in with colour. Allow the person freedom to experiment with colour as well as time and space to enjoy his colouring adventure. His work can be used as a conversational and reminiscing tool.

PAINTING TO MUSIC

Spread a large sheet of paper between the patient and
you. Put on some soft music and close your eyes for a
moment or two to get the feel of the sound and rhythm
Ask the patient to do the same. Open your eyes and
draw the music as you hear it. Or you can each draw
facial expression showing how the music made you
feel.

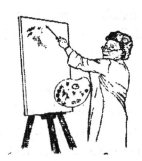

TRACING

Trace your hand or foot on a piece of paper and ask th
patient to draw in fingernails. Or draw the outline of
head and ask the patient to fill in the eyes, nose and
mouth. These activities encourage an awareness of
body parts and their relation to one another.

COMPLETE THE PICTURE

Draw a shape on a piece of paper. Pass it to the patien
and ask him to add something. Take it back and add
something else yourself. Continue passing the picture
back and forth and discuss whatever emerges.

HOBBIES

Many patients can still engage in hobbies such as sewing, pottery and woodwork during the early stages of the disease while motor abilities are relatively unimpaired. As the disease advances however, cognitive functions begin to decline and patients soon find it difficult to work out, for example, how a screwdriver works or how to follow a sewing pattern. The tendency is for people to drop hobbies once difficulties set in. If, however, the tasks are simplified, hobbies can bring pleasure well into the disease.

The key is to reduce the hobby to its simplest terms. If, for example, the patient has enjoyed pottery all her life, give her a ball of clay to knead. The tactile experience of working with clay will have pleasant associations and will give rise to a feeling of sensory familiarity.

Hobby materials must be made simple and safe. Sharp or pointed tools such as sewing needles or knives can be replaced with harmless substitutes. A metal hammer can be replaced with a wooden mallet; a plastic shovel may work just as well as a metal trowel.

When the patient can no longer perform even a simple version of a former hobby, there are still ways to maintain her interest. Someone who can no longer play the guitar, for example, may still enjoy listening to recordings. A patient who can no longer sew may still enjoy going to craft shows and fingering through exhibits. This kind of involvement kindles memories and provides sensory satisfaction.

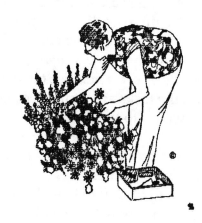

VISITORS

Visits from close friends and family members are vitally important. They are an antidote to the loneliness and isolation that often ensue as a result of Alzheimer's disease and link both patient and care-giver with the community. When it is not possible for old friends to visit in person, they can keep in touch by making occasional phone calls and sending cards and letters.

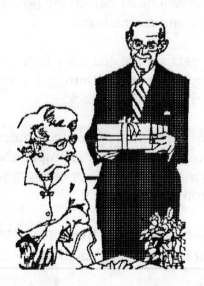

Visits should be kept calm and uncomplicated. Short one-to-one social calls are best. Visits by more than a few people at a time are confusing as patients have difficulty recognising people and keeping up with shifts in conversation.

71

GUIDELINES FOR VISITS

The following steps will help ensure successful visits.

- Ask visitors to come for short visits.

- If visitors are totally unfamiliar with the disease, give them something to read beforehand. Exceller brochures are available from the Alzheimer's Disease Societies.

- Brief visitors on the patient's condition and point out subjects that are still of interest to her.

- Reserve a quiet part of the house for visits. Limit noise and distractions.

- Suggest simple activities for the visit: browsing through a photo album, going for a short walk, or sharing a special snack.

- Give the visitor tips for communicating with the patient. Suggest, for example, that she avoid askin too many questions or changing the topic of conve sation too frequently.

- Make sure you let the person know how much the visit has meant to you both.

HUMOUR

Many patients retain a hearty sense of humour despite the disease process. This can be capitalised on. Laughing sets off biological processes that improve health by increasing the blood flow to the brain and the oxygen level. Laughing releases endorphins into the brain. This releases stress and tension and creates a natural high.

Do what you can to bring laughter into the patient's life and bring out her sense of fun. In your everyday interactions, make use of little jokes and pleasantries. Reminisce over amusing events. Tell an amusing anecdote. These will help lighten the atmosphere and will make you both feel better.

Have an occasional 'comedy hour'. Videotapes of old comedies by the Marx Brothers, Lucille Ball and Charlie Chaplin will get the laughter juices flowing. Find out when old radio shows are being repeated. The short story lines of these old shows make ideal listening for those with short attention spans.

Read extracts from books of humour. See if you can find a good book of jokes in the library. Share newspaper cartoons such as Andy Capp and Charlie Brown, which have been around for many years. The belly laughs which result will erase all trace of depression and painful feelings.

OUTINGS

Short outdoor trips are stimulating and provide a sociable and healthy change of scene. Outdoor trips also aid in reality orientation, keeping patients abreast with changes in the community such as new shopping malls, community centres or housing estates.

A weekly visit to the local day care centre adds variety to the patient's social life and exposes her to new friends and activities. Talk to the director about having the patient attend for lunch or participate in the activity programme. Even a short weekly visit will help lessen the patient's isolation and give you some time for yourself.

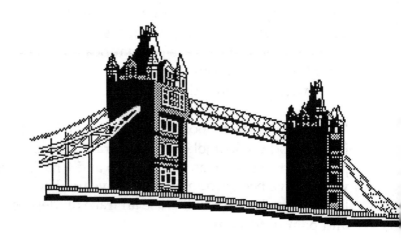

The patient may be able to go shopping for groceries with you occasionally and may be able to select some favourite items. Trips to the park are often popular and therapeutic, providing fresh air and contact with nature. Some patients enjoy eating out in a quiet restaurant occasionally, especially in the early stages of the disease. Visits can also be made to the homes of friends and relatives, or, if possible, to the patient's former office or workplace. Make sure that places to be visited are stress-free and quiet.

A change of scene, no matter how apparently suitable, can still increase confusion and anxiety. Reassure the patient frequently and cut the outing short if he becomes unduly agitated.

OTHER PLACES TO VISIT :
museum
concert
library
grandchild's school
art gallery
church
theatre
countryside
zoo
historical landmarks

PETS

People with Alzheimer's disease often relate very well to pets. Pets offer the kind of unconditional acceptance that people with Alzheimer's crave. They provide companionship and affection as well as tactile comfort. The physical contact and soft sensations have a relaxing effect. Pets offer an opportunity for play and provide a welcome distraction from problems. They encourage physical exercise and social interaction. Relating to a a pet is often less stressful for the patient than human interaction.

If you already have a pet, try to create situations in which the patient is doing the caring. Caring for a pet provides the patient with an outlet for his need to nurture. Walking the pet, washing, stroking, caressing and feeding it under supervision — all make the patient feel needed and useful.

GETTING A NEW PET

There are many considerations to make in deciding to get a pet. Factors such as expense, who will care for the pet, discipline and the choice of pet have to be weighed carefully. Puppies are usually the most popular. Next line are kittens, followed by rabbits. Many patients enjoy handling and caressing small, furry rodents such as hamsters, gerbils, and white mice. Make sure you choose a pet with a very pleasant disposition.

PROVIDING ACCESS TO PETS

Families under stress may find that the discipline and attention that a new pet demands may be too disruptive. If this is the case, an aquarium with some small fish, or a bird, are fair substitutes. You can also try taking the patient to the park to feed the ducks or to a local pet shop where he might be able to hold a kitten or puppy.

You may have a friend whose pet you can borrow or visit on occasion if you have none of your own. People who must keep their pet locked up all day are often receptive to visiting arrangements. Also worth looking into are "visiting pet" programmes offered by local veterinary associations. These organisations often sponsor and help arrange visits from pets to the homes of elderly persons. They usually have lists of local pet owners on file who are willing to participate in such programmes. In some day care centres, volunteers make arrangements with the local RSPCA to bring dogs and cats to the centre so that the patients can be entertained and the animals exercised.

Perhaps the easiest and most stress-free way to provide contact with pets is through installing a birdfeeder. A feeder perch can be attached outside the window of the patient's room or a hanging bird feeder can be located nearby. The person can be encouraged to fill the feeder in the morning and will enjoy watching the birds as they come and go during the seasons.

REALITY ORIENTATION

Simple activities can be used to help the patient stay in touch with her surroundings. These activities are based on reality orientation—a technique for reducing confusion by providing patients with reality-based information such as their name, whereabouts and the time.

A reality orientation bulletin board, such as the one illustrated below, can be used to post information and the patient can be encouraged to fill in the board daily. A large calendar might be placed on the wall and the patient asked to tear off each day's date. This helps orientate her to the time of year.

Sunnyside Home, Devonshire	
Today is	Monday
The date is	March 1st 1991
The weather is	warm and sunny
The next holiday is	St. Patrick's Day

Memory aids are a central part of reality orientation. All of us resort to memory aids of one kind or another in our everyday lives. Wrist watches, clocks, calendars, lists and notes are popular examples. The need for memory aids is so much greater among those with Alzheimer's disease.

Family photographs can be used to keep patients orientated to current relationships. Pictures taken at celebrations and outings can be used to help people maintain awareness of events, places and people. Ask questions such as "Who is the gentleman to your right in the photo?" or "Tell me about this picture of your niece." Awareness of current events, fashions and food prices can be enhanced by the use of newspapers.

RO can be used to address specific orientation problems. Some patients, for example, cannot remember their own address and feel a lot of anxiety as a result. Help her print her address on an index card and encourage her to consult it when she needs this information.

OTHER ACTIVITIES

- Cut out newspaper articles and pictures for discussion. The "local" section of the paper will be particularly relevant as well as the local news.

- Help the patient make cards to send to family and friends at birthdays and holidays.

- Write out the day's activities and encourage the patient to tick off each activity as they are completed.

- Show pictures of familiar everyday objects and food to the patient and ask her to tell you about them.

SELF-CARE ACTIVITIES

Once the patient starts experiencing difficulties with self-care activities, the tendency is for the care-giver to step in and take over. This is a natural reaction as it saves time. However, patients are likely to lose the abilities they don't use. It is more helpful if you can avoid taking over and instead help the patient help himself.

Try simplifying self-care activities and allowing the patient independence for as long as possible. This builds self-esteem, keeps the patient in touch with his appearance and builds body awareness.

DRESSING

Dressing can be made into a simple, failure-free activit by following these steps:

- To make the selection of clothes easier, put away out-of-season clothes or articles that are seldom worn.

- Label dressing table drawers clearly to remind the person what is in them.

- Lay out articles of clothing in the order they are intended to be put on.

- Simplify clothing: replace buttons, snaps, hooks, zippers and belt buckles with Velcro tape. Make sure the person has slip-on shoes instead of shoes with laces. Jogging bottoms or tracksuits are good alternatives for the person who has difficulty dressing.

GROOMING

Help the patient to look attractive and maintain a positive self-image. Women enjoy receiving manicures and having make-up applied. They can participate by choosing the colours of nail polish, lipstick and eye shadow and selecting their own perfume. Try to find a suitable hairstyle which is easy to care for. Men will enjoy an occasional trip to the barber. Having a regular haircut and shave lifts the spirits and gives men pride in their appearance.

MEALTIMES

Patients can continue to feed themselves for longer if mealtimes are simplified. There are a number of things you can do to make eating easier for your relative and more pleasant for you. Some involve the way meals are served and others involve the food eaten. Here are some suggestions.

- Reduce distractions and noise during mealtimes.

- Serve only one food at a time.

- Serve finger foods which are easy to manage. Vegetables, fruits, sandwiches and chips are some examples.

- Use helpful devices such as a sectioned plate with high sides or a "scoop dish".

- The table setting should be simple, with just what is needed for eating. The table cloth should be a solid colour, with no pattern.

SENSORY STIMULATION

Many patients are very withdrawn, particularly in the later stages of the disease. Simple activities can be used to stimulate the senses and bring patients out of their isolation.

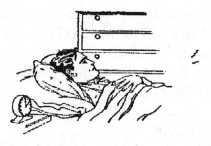

MASSAGE

Touch is perhaps the most eloquent communication tool we have. During the day, there are many opportunities for expressing affection through a hug, a stroke, or a handshake. Each gesture is a gentle reminder to the person that you are present to help, comfort and guide her.

Patients are usually very receptive to the healing impact of a slow, gentle and firm massage. From five to ten minutes is long enough as the patient's attention span is short. Start on the back using circular stroking motions and proceed to the arms. Use long firm strokes and keep in mind that many older people are tender and fragile. Be very gentle and don't use any unfamiliar pounding motions. Use warm oil and if the person's skin is dry, use a moisturing emollient. End at the torso, legs and feet.

BACK RUB

Much tension can accumulate in the neck and shoulder area of people who are sedentary. You can gently rub away the tension in this area in the evenings while viewing a television programme, after dinner or before bed. As you do so, take time to find out about any worries or concerns the person has.

HAND MASSAGE

This is a loving way to communicate. Gently rub a few drops of Vitamin E oil into the patient's hands talking to her as you do so. Massage each hand gently. As you do so, talk gently with her or hum special tune.

FOOT SOAK

A foot soak can be a soothing night-time ritual an an effective way to close the day. Play gentle background music as you cradle each foot in the comfort of a soft solution of water and epsom salts. Water softens the skin, refreshes the feet and removes residues of dead skin. Oil and massage eacl foot afterwards and wrap in a warm towel. Dust between the toes with baby powder. The loving atmosphere created will help the patient to open up and confide in you.

ACTIVITIES INVOLVING SMELL

The sense of smell is often quite impaired in Alzheimer's disease. It can be gently stimulated b providing odours that are related to the person's life. Scents revive memories and have strong associations for people. The smell of baked bread or a turkey cooking, for example, remind us of family times, while the smell of freshly turned soil makes us think of time spent in the country.

Help people remember a pleasant time or experience in their lives through fragrances. When choosing scents, make sure they are somehow related to the individual and his past. Spices and herbs might work well for a former cook, while permanent waving solution would have stronger associations for a former beautician.

Tell the patient you have chosen a scent which she might remember from her childhood, job or growing up years. Let her smell the item and engage her through touch and conversation. Withdrawn persons may respond with only a faint smile, but the scent can trigger memories and pleasant thoughts that last for hours.

ACTIVITIES INVOLVING TASTE

Taste is closely linked with the sense of smell. Try to stimulate the patient's sense of taste with various foods and liquids. These can be presented in small medicine cups. This activity can lead to a discussion about favourite foods, memories of food in the old days and what foods aren't available now.

ACTIVITIES INVOLVING SOUND

Sounds can be used to trigger memories or to make the patient aware of people and events in her surroundings. Make tape recordings of a variety of sounds. Use sounds that are personally relevant to the individual or that are connected with the season or location. The sound of a train whistle sounding would have strong associations for a former railway guard. A former school teacher might relate to the sound of a school bell ringing, while a farmer would probably respond to the sound of a dog barking or a cock crowing.

Tell the patient you have something for her to listen to and let her share whatever associations come up. Some patients are so withdrawn that they may not respond verbally. Don't see this as a failure.

ACTIVITIES INVOLVING SIGHT

The sense of sight can be stimulated through looking at common everyday objects, such as a cup, teapot, mirror, door knob or broom. These items can be discussed and their use demonstrated. Photographs of family, friends and nature are also a rich source of stimulation and potential discussion.

SPIRITUAL ACTIVITIES

Many patients find great comfort and strength in their religion as they become frail. Do what you can to help the patient pursue her beliefs and practices. Join her in saying grace before meals, if this has been her practice. Make devotional and religious reading materials available to her and read her short passages or extracts. Find out what religious resources are close to your home or nursing home and avail of these.

The homebound patient may be able to listen to church services on radio or television. Some churches even record their services and cassette tapes of these are available for the asking. Perhaps the local minister, priest or rabbi could visit the patient at home. Many church or synagogue members will also extend this courtesy, if asked.

Perhaps the patient can do something for the church to support the feeling of belonging. Simple activities such as repairing hymnals, arranging flowers, stapling newsletters, or folding programmes might be possible.

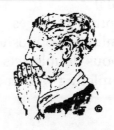

WORD GAMES

Things learned and remembered in childhood can ofte
be easily recalled by persons with Alzheimer's disease
The alphabet, counting numbers and nursery rhymes
are some examples. The major capital cities, the prime
ministers, the colours and even poetry, (memorized as
long as a half century before!) may also be recited
effortlessly.

Word games based on recall of this kind are often
popular with Alzheimer patients. For example, you ca
supply the first part of an old proverb and let the patient fill in the missing part. Once cued in this way, h
can experience the success of completing the proverb.
Reciting an old nursery rhyme after being "cued" with
the opening line will provide the same kind of satisfac
tion.

Make a list of the kinds of things people memorize ov
the years and invent simple word games based on thes
categories. Here are some examples.

- Prayers (The Lords Prayer and Grace Before
  Meals)
- Scripture passages
- Naming the opposite (black and white)
- Famous double acts
- Completing well known phrases

FAMILY ACTIVITIES

Being included in family events gives the person with A.D. a much needed sense of belonging. Whenever you can, set a place for the patient at the table during family meals. Let her participate in simple household chores. The feeling of doing her part and contributing in some way will mean a lot to her.

Let patients celebrate holidays with their families. Keep them abreast of family news. Invite them to childrens' birthday parties and special events. If possible, include them in small social gatherings throughout the year.

When the family clan is together, make time for sharing through simple activities. You may want to designate one evening a week as family night and have one or two relatives visit. Try to make family night the same each week so that family members will keep that night free when making individual plans. Here are some special activities you can share.

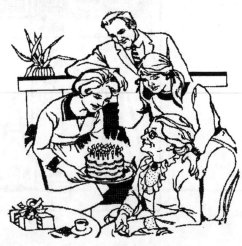

LIFE COLLAGE

Involve the patient in making his own life collage.
can include a written biographical sketch
mentioning his former occupation, achievements
and interests. Photos of family and friends and
pictures of places lived in can be included. Hang
the collage in an obvious part of the patient's room
It will provide a good topic of conversation for
visitors who are often unsure of what to talk abou

Materials Needed for Life Collage:

- Large sheet of mounting board
- Sticky Tape
- Safety Scissors
- Written biographical sketch /family tree
- Photographs

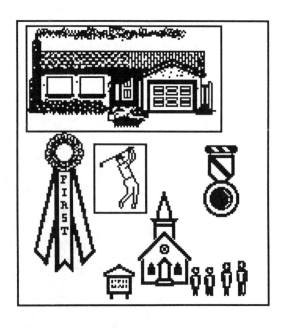

MAKE A MEMORY BOOK

A memory book can provide a written and pictorial record of the patient's life. It can be compiled with the help of the patient and at a pace conducive to reminiscing.

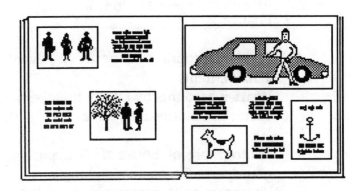

Family members at all levels can become involved, working with the patient and slowly piecing together the highlights of his life. Pictures, headlines and news items from old newspapers and magazines can be pasted in where appropriate, to put the patient's life in context.

The local library or historical society may have additional material which would help to illustrate what was happening locally during the patient's life. If there are children in the family, leafing through the memory book with the patient will help them to share something from his past. On completion, the memory book will provide the patient with hours of passive entertainment.

Materials needed for memory book :

- Large spiral notebook or scrapbook
  Felt tipped pens or crayons
  Sticky Tape
  Old newspapers
  Magazines and catalogues
  Postcards

- Written accounts of experiences, events and achievements
  Written accounts by family members of special memories they have of the patient

- Photographs of house of birth, parents, grandparents, cousins, siblings etc.
  Photographs of memorable moments: graduation, wedding, birth of children, retirement etc.

MAKE A MEMORY BOX

Help the patient to make a memory box consisting of objects from his past. Hunt for early "junk" in attics, basements and store-rooms. Any memorabilia from the patient's life will probably be useful—trophies, autograph books, postcards, stamp albums, report cards, school books, even diaries and letters belonging to the patient. The memory box can include very old items from the patient's childhood.

The memory box can be placed beside the patient's chair, and will provide a stimulus for discussion.

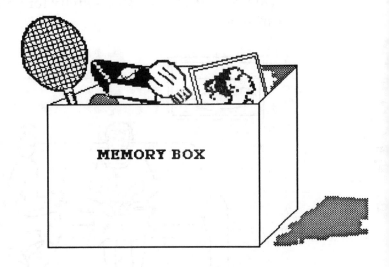

Family members can pay attention to what stimulates his curiosity most to get clues for further themes for conversation. By exploring the memory box with their relative, children can learn more about "the old days."

The memory box provides a wonderful focus for conversation for visitors who can draw on it to talk about the past. Friends may even be able to add old photographs and various knick-knacks when they visit. For the patient who is conscious of his memory loss, the memory box makes visits from friends easier by providing a conversation piece.

PHOTO ALBUM

Old photographs are a wonderful resource for reminiscence and browsing through a photo album will provide an enjoyable activity for patient and care-giver.

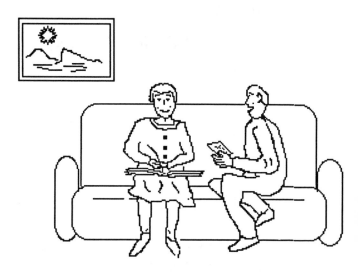

The patient's history or that of the family can be pieced together pictorially using family photo albums. Families often label photos to help the patient remember relatives and close friends. Learn which photos are most important to the patient so he can carry them around in a pocket if he wishes. As conversation pieces, photos are excellent.

HOME MOVIES AND SLIDES

Old home movies, taken when family members were younger, provide an excellent stimulus for reminiscence and "then" and "now" comparisons. Likewise, slides of places and people once familiar to the patient can evoke memories of very distant times. Families which have these visual materials should recognize their usefulness in eliciting memories.

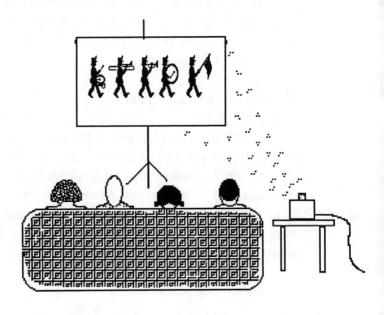

VCR equipment gives an opportunity for viewing films at opportune times without commercial interruptions and videos of favourite old-time movies could be hired occasionally. A special family night for viewing movies and slides can be arranged every so often.

RECORDING A FAMILY AUDIO TAPE

Create a 20 minute audio history of your relative's life. Make it conversational, lively and brief. Imagine the person sitting in front of you as you speak and talk directly to him. Begin by saying..."your name is ...you live at...and your telephone number is...You live with me, Mary at... (repeat the address)". Then present a brief history of his life including achievements or special honours. Put the emphasis on praising him and his good traits. Include some humour and anecdotes. Conclude by repeating his name and address. Listening to this tape daily will reinforce reality for the patient and improve his self-esteem.

MAKING A FAMILY VIDEO

Family members can make video tapes of their families and these make entertaining viewing. They can speak directly to the patient, wave at him and take him on a tour of their homes. They can tell him they love him and miss him and look forward to seeing him again. Looking at the tape will give the patient a feeling of well-being and security and the care-giver will have a brief respite to complete household tasks.

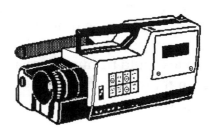

SIMPLE GAMES

There are many simple parlour games which the A.D. patient may be able to play. Games should be short and not demand much concentration.

NUMBER BINGO

A simplified version of Bingo with only the numbers 1 to 12 can be played to bring the game within the confused person's memory span. Here, each person has a card with 4-6 numbers in large, easy-to-read format.

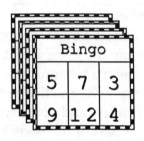

PICTURE BINGO

In picture bingo each person has a card with less than five easily identifiable pictures on it. The more personally relevant the pictures are, the better. The winner is the first to match all his pictures.

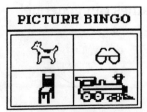

MONEY BINGO
Some patients may be able to play Money Bingo
where coins are matched with their money values.

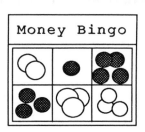

CHARADES
Word games can be played with letter cards, turning up say the letter E and asking the patient to
name a word beginning with it. A game of cha-
rades can give practice in word-finding, body part
identification and social interaction. For example,
"name a part of the body beginning with E."

PAPER AND PENCIL GAMES
Some patients will remember how to play simple
children's games such as Hangman, Connect the
Dots, Squares, or Noughts and Crosses. Other paper-
and-pencil games are legion. For example, draw a
picture of a face and have the patient add eyes and
nose. You will be surprised at how much fun these
games can generate!

CARD GAMES

Patients may have played simple card games such as Memory, Go Fish and War in their younger days. Black jack, poker, roulette, and other card games can still be played by many in the early stages of the disease. The patient will enjoy the familiar card-playing scene and it will stimulate memory recall. You can simplify the process by obtaining cards with large face numbers. Keep in mind that players will probably require assistance in making certain decisions. Keep the group small, go slowly and give help generously.

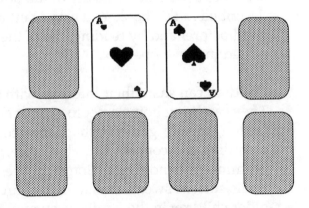

ACTIVITIES INVOLVING CHILDREN

With their spontaneity and uninhibited ways, young children are often a source of joy to the Alzheimer's patient. Children tend to have access to healing energies not available to the average adult. You can capitalize on this by inviting your local school to send children to visit your day-care centre.

In the home, the playful presence of children can do much to lighten the atmosphere and bring a sense of fun to the patient's life. Children can take part in the activities above and in many of the other activities described in this book. You may want to prepare the child beforehand by reading one of the books suggested in the Appendix.

Children can share their interests with the patient. They can bring home a pet to visit or share a stamp collection, book or game. Perhaps they could share a tape recording of a concert, church service, school programme or band recital. Some children enjoy bringing treats such as sweets or snacks to share. If there are older children in the family, they may be able to help the patient maintain ties with friends by reading cards and letters for her and helping her make phone calls.

REMINISCENCE

Reviewing the past is a universal process that occurs most frequently in later life. Many elderly people have vivid memories of their past and can recall life events with remarkable clarity. People with profound memory loss often enjoy recounting their life stories to anyone who is willing to listen. Families may have difficulty in understanding how an Alzheimer's relative who cannot remember his own age or what he had for his last meal, can still recount a story from his childhood in detail. The reason has to do with the nature of memory loss in the disease. Loss of memory for recent events is usually profound, so that individuals may have difficulty remembering the previous sentence in a conversation, or the story line of a television film. But long-term memory, that is memory of events in the distant past, may remain relatively intact, particularly throughout the early stages of the disease.

Group reminiscence sessions are now used in many nursing homes and day-care facilities which specialize in the care of victims of Alzheimer's disease. They provide participants with an opportunity to relive some of the past experiences of their lives. Families too can use reminiscence on a one-to-one basis with their memory-impaired relative at home (this was explored under the section **Family Activities**).

Talking about the past calls upon the patient's interests or skills of long ago and in so doing, validates his life contributions, interests and feelings. The focus on validation is central to reminiscence. It helps acknowledge the person the patient was and continues to be, despite the disease process.

In many reminiscence discussions, use is made of old items such as books, pictures and records to provoke memories. Memorabilia which have lain unused for years assume a new importance when they are used for reminiscence.

REMINISCENCE DISCUSSIONS

Reminiscing feels safe for people with Alzheimer's disease because they are more in control when talking about the past. Remember though, that reminiscing with your relative is <u>not</u> the same as encouraging him to live in the past. The following guidelines are worth remembering as you reminisce together.

- Help keep facts accurate by relating them to the past as opposed to the present.

- Discuss topics in a quiet, unhurried way, giving the patient ample time to respond.

- Give cues and prompts where necessary.

- Use a tangible focus for each topic—something concrete that the patient can see such as a photograph or souvenir. This will help to prompt memories and will remind tthe patient of what the conversation is about.

THEMES FOR REMINISCENCE

Build a bank of themes for reminiscence. From the following suggestions, select those which the patient can relate to best.

HOME
Where was your first home ? Did you move often? Why? What was your favourite house?

SCHOOL
Where did you attend your first school ? What was the school like? Who taught you ? Who was your favourite teacher? What was your favourite subject?

PETS
Did you ever have a pet? What did you call it? How did you decide on its name? Would you like to have a pet now? (Show pictures of popular pets)

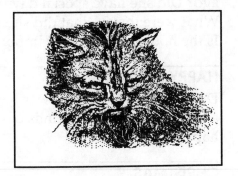

NAMES
Do you recall the names of childhood friends? Who gave you your name—your mother or father? Is there a special name you would like to have been called by? What is your favourite name? What

names don't you like? Why?

PASTIMES
What was your favourite pastime ? Did you ever go fishing? Sailing ? Who went with you ? Where did you go ?

SPORTS
Did you have a favourite sport? What teams did you follow? Who were the stars?

HOSPITAL
Were you ever in hospital? Why? How much did it cost in the old days? Did you try out home remedies before going to hospital? Are there any special nurses or doctors you recall from that time?

HOUSEKEEPING
How was the housewife's week organised long ago? Did she have special days for certain chores? What were they? What did she use as an iron? Is the housewife's role as important nowadays?

HAPPY DAYS
Do you recall a day that was happier than all others? Describe it. What kinds of things make you happy now?

CHRISTMAS
How did you celebrate Christmas when you were a child? Was it a special holiday for you? What was your favourite Christmas game? Did you ever go to a fancy-dress Christmas ball?

HOLIDAYS

What was your most memorable holiday? Who did you go with? Tell me about some funny happenings. (Use pictures, photos, posters and brochures.)

BOOKS

Tell me about your favourite books. What books do you like to look at now? Did you read Shakespeare when you were young? Did you like mysteries?

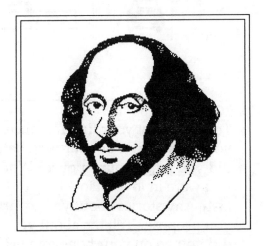

FOOD

Do you have a favourite food? What kind of food did you eat during the war? Tell me what your ideal meal would consist of.

TELEVISION

Tell me about your first TV. What were your favourite programmes? Can you name the personalities? What was home life like before TV?

TRANSPORT

What special transport did you use growing up?
Did you drive, own a car, have a bike? What kind
was your first car? Pictures of various modes of
transport will aid discussions.

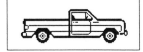

ROMANCE

Tell me about your first romance. Do you recall
your first dance or your first date. How
did you meet your spouse? When did you know
you were in love? How long did your engagement
last? Any stories about your courtship? How did
you propose? Tell me about your wedding. Where
did you go on your honeymoon?

CHILDREN

At what age did you have your first child? How
did you decide on the name? Tell me about some of
the happy times. What about the hard times?

GIFTS

Were you ever given a gift that you have always
treasured? Why was it special? Describe some gifts
you have given. Do you still have it?

WORK

What jobs did you have? Do you recall spending your first week's or month's earnings? Who worked with you? What jobs did members of your family do?

PRICES

Discuss changes in the cost of living over the years. Show price lists. Many elderly people in nursing homes may be shocked at the price increases in foods such as milk, sugar and tea. Find out how much a haircut cost in the old days or how much it cost to go to the cinema. How much did it cost to buy a house or a car, or to have a tooth extracted?

THE WAR

What age were you when it began? What job did you have? What are your memories of working conditions at that time? How was morale in your community? Did you go to war?

FASHIONS

Were you fashion-conscious? What type of clothes did you like to wear? Did you have a choice or did you wear hand-me-downs? Were hats popular in your day? What do your think of the way people dress today? What has been your favourite fashion of all time?

APPENDIX A

SUGGESTED READING FOR CARE-GIVERS

The 36 Hour Day by Mace, N & Rabins, P
This is an excellent readable explanation of many prob
lem behaviours and symptoms in Alzheimer's disease
Highlighted are the emotional implications for the
spouse and adult child, as well as the importance of
supportive help from relatives, friends, self-help
groups, and professional groups. Also dealt with are
legal, financial and placement issues that every family
must face. Essentially directed at the family, this book
also a useful guide for professionals.
Available from: Age Concern England, Astral House,
1268 London Road, London SW16 4EJ

**Caring for the Person with Dementia - A Guide for
Families and Other Carers.**
Alzheimer's Disease Society, 158-160 Balham High
Road, London SW12 9BN

**Coping With Caring - A Guide to Identifying and
Supporting an Elderly Person with Dementia** by Dr.
Brian Lodge
Available from: MIND Mail Order Service, 4th Floor,
24-32 Stephenson Way, London NW1 2HD

APPENDIX B

VIDEOS FOR CARE-GIVERS

Excellent films, videos, slides and training packs are available from the Scottish Central Film Library, 74 Victoria Crescent, Dowanhill, Glasgow G12 9JG or from the Alzheimer's Disease Society in London, or Alzheimer's Scotland in Edinburgh. All of these videos are on the VHS system and are copyright material. They are available for loan or hire.

Contact: **Alzheimer's Disease Society,** 158-160 Balham High Road, London SW12 9BN**, or Alzheimer's Scotland,** 33 Castle Street, Edinburgh EH2 3DN for a list of videos for hire and for further information.

Where is the Key? An hour long authorised BBC videotape of a successful television drama which documents the problems facing both patient and care-giver.

Suffer the Carers A video about self-help groups. Made by the Alzheimer's Society with Siddartha Films, it illustrates how the self-help group can support the sufferer and carer. 35 minutes

Mental Confusion and the Elderly A four-part video series on the diagnosis of dementia and its managment in the community and institution.

APPENDIX C
ACTIVITY RESOURCES

Many of the following activity resources have been specially designed with the Alzheimer's patient in mind. They have few, large, easily-handled pieces and the pictures are simple and easily recognisable. These and many other resources are available from:
Winslow Press, Telford Road, Bicester,Oxon, OX6 OT

SEQUENCING

Basic Sequences Everyday easily identified activities are the hallmark of this superb set. Sixteen 3-card sequences show people performing common everyday sequentially-related actions. These include making a telephone call, ironing clothes, feeding a dog, shaving and sewing. 01-673

Social Sequences From cooking an omelette to going the doctor or from visiting a library to having a bath, these multi-card sets develop social skills, reasoning and left to right sequencing. 64 clear and colourful cards each measuring 70 x 105mm. 30-445

RING BOARD

Arm exercise, distance judgement and hand/eye coordination are all encouraged with this superb and safe game. The board is almost 43cm high and holds 1 numbered hooks. Six rubber rings are supplied. Individuals, pairs or teams will all enjoy this game.

BINGO

The bingo shutter tray offers single -line, short game bingo. It has large, easy-to-see numbers and can be used instead of a bingo card. It's an ideal resource for people who have difficulty in manipulating a marker for checking. The plastic shutters are pulled across when the number is called. 54-556

PUZZLES

Stand-up Jigsaws Unique limewood jigsaw puzzles of animals designed to stand up when pieced together. This whole new dimension in jigsaws, with few and large easy-to-handle pieces, is especially suited to elderly confused people. 44-496

Inset Puzzle Pack The large easy-to-grip knobs and the strong construction make this Inset Puzzle Pack a useful manipulative activity. Contoured for rigid hands, these pegs help develop fine motor control. The shoulder on each peg insures a positive stop when inserted into the pegboard. 83-766

SORTING

Everyday Objects (ColorCards) These carefully selected domestic objects have been arranged in six categories, each with a colour-coded background. The cards can be used for discussion or can be shuffled and used as a sorting activity.

REMINISCENCE

Reminiscing This game provides memories of past events, trends, TV and films etc. from the 1950s to the 1980s. Players are prompted to remember thoughts and feelings from their personal past, including recent decades. 19-1535

Famous Faces A particularly stimulating photc pack containing 40 well-known personalities who achieved fame between the years 1920 anc 1960. Taken from the world of sport, politics ar entertainment, they are faces that will live forever—Louis Armstrong, Stanley Matthews, Winston Churchill and many more. A useful manual accompanies the pack, giving a brief biography of each celebrity. Armed with these personal details and interesting anecdotes, gro leaders should find it much easier to stimulate discussion and revive many associated memories. 01-141

MUSIC

Music of Yesteryear This careful selection of 1: tapes provides music for individual and group listening. They can be used as background mu. to evoke nostalgic memories of the past. A balanced selection is provided from wartime memories stirred by Vera Lynn to memories ol happier times evoked by the hits of the thirties These 12 music cassettes are packaged in a useful carrying case. 07-135

APPENDIX D

USEFUL ORGANISATIONS

The following organisations provide family members and caregivers with information about Alzheimer's disease, care options and services. Contact your national Alzheimer's Society and get on their newsletter mailing list. They may also be able to put you in contact with a local branch and support group.

Alzheimer's Disease Society
158-160 Balham High Road
London SW12 9BN
England

Alzheimer's Scotland
33 Castle Street
Edinburgh, EH2 3DN
Scotland
24-hour Dementia Helpline: 031-220 6155 for information and support

Alzheimer's Society of Ireland
St. John of God Hospital
Stillorgan
Co. Dublin
Ireland

Alzheimerforeningen
Sankt Lukas Vej 13
2900 Hellerup
Denmark

Alzheimer's Organisation of Finland
Tøpeliuksenkatu 17C
00250 Helsinki
Finland

France Alzheimer
49 rue Mirabeau
75016 Paris
France

Deutsche Alzheimer's Gesel schaft
Mauerkircher Strasse 21
Mohlstrasse 26
8000 München 80 (9)
Germany

Associazione Italiana Malattia di Alzheimer
Sezione di Milano
Via Marino 7
I+20121 Milano
Italy

Alzheimerföreningen
Sunnanvag 14S
S-22226 Lund
Sweden

Alzheimer Stichting
J.F. Kennedylann 99
3921 GB Bunnih
PO Box 100
3900CC Bunnih
Netherlands

Alzheimer's Association (Australia)
PO Box 51
North Ryde
New South Wales 2113
Australia

Alzheimer Society of Canada
1320 Yonge Street, Suite 302
Toronto
Ontario M4T 1X2
Canada

Mexican Alzheiemer's Association
Irlanda 124
Col. Parque San Andrezs Coyoacan
Mexico 21, D.F. 04040

ADARDS N.Z. Inc
Box 2808
Christchurch
New Zealand

Alzheimer's Association
PO Box 81183
Parkhurst
Johannesburg 2120
South Africa